HERBS FOR HEALTHY HAIR

Describes twenty herbs that have proved particularly beneficial for hair care. Includes shampoos, tonics, conditioners and rinses, as well as remedies for helping deal with specific problems such as baldness, premature greying, dry, greasy, or fading hair.

By the same author
FREE FOR ALL
HERBAL TEAS FOR HEALTH AND HEALING

In this series
HERBS AND FRUIT FOR SLIMMERS
HERBS AND FRUIT FOR VITAMINS
HERBS FOR ACIDITY AND GASTRIC ULCERS
HERBS FOR FIRST-AID AND MINOR
   AILMENTS
HERBS TO HELP YOU SLEEP

HERBS
FOR
HEALTHY HAIR

by
CERES

Drawings by Alison Ross

THORSONS PUBLISHERS LIMITED
Wellingborough, Northamptonshire

First published 1977

ISBN 0 7225 0375 X

Photoset by Specialised Offset Services Ltd, Liverpool and Printed and bound in Great Britain by Weatherby Woolnough, Wellingborough, Northamptonshire

CONTENTS

INTRODUCTION

At all stages of our lives, from childhood to old age, a head of lively and glossy hair must surely be one of the most admirable outward signs of a healthy body and mind.

There may be those who disagree with this statement, but I believe that the hair is the external 'barometer of our inward condition' and it is surprising how few people seem to have plenty of really lustrous locks. Those who do are usually well-balanced and stable people with a happy and even outlook on life, who seldom suffer illness.

Nowadays there seems to be almost a fetish about having ultra-clean hair and I am inclined to think that there can be too much hair-washing. It depends, of course, on the circumstances and on the type of shampoo that is used, and there are some herbal recipes which can easily be made at home which really ought to be harmless even if used frequently.

My family pick and use herbs from the garden for shampoos. We put a handful of young Nettles (picked with gloves on), a few branch-tips of Rosemary, Southernwood and Sage, and a few leaves of Yarrow and some stripped-off Lavender or a few drops of Lavender oil, into a saucepan and simmer them in a quart of water for ten or fifteen minutes. The herbs are then strained off and a teacupful (our water is hard so you may need less) of shredded Castile Soap is stirred in with a wooden spoon until it is melted. This makes plenty for four of us, but it should be used fresh and it is simple to make individual half-pint shampoos by cutting down the ingredients proportionally. The herbs, of course, can be varied depending upon the scent preferred or the particular need or availability of the moment.

If you have a source of clean rain water that can be filtered and boiled to use as a basis for a final rinse, it is far kinder and more softening to the hair than most tap water.

But even with the careful use of harmless shampoos plus a good daily stimulating brushing of the hair to remove dust and loose hairs and also to massage the scalp (and, by the way, do avoid nylon brushes and sharp-toothed combs which can damage both hair and scalp), there can still be hair problems. Few older people seem to be without some hair difficulties which, on the whole, I would put down to dietary deficiencies or the use of harsh detergents and solutions by most hairdressers.

Hereditary baldness is something that creeps up on many men and however much trouble they take to avoid it, it seems impossible to overcome. Women too have their trials, in that more and more of them are suffering from premature greying of the hair.

But, herbalists say, both processes can be halted! Or at least hindered! Let me take baldness first. Many of the old recipes recommend the juice of Nettles, either fresh or from a professionally prepared tincture. It is easy enough to express Nettle juice (with a juicer) yourself and well worth a try to see if it stimulates fresh hair-growth. Try it diluted at first and use it to brush and comb through remaining hair and into the scalp. The exact strength should be determined by experimenting but I would start by putting a teaspoonful of neat juice into a cup of water and seeing how it affects your head. As it contains the contents of the stinging hairs of the plant, Nettle juice can be an irritant if used too strong, so it is wise to start carefully.

Yarrow is a traditional 'baldwort' or hair-restorer and there are plenty of other suggested cures, including the drastic idea of rubbing a cut onion into the scalp daily. This is not to be recommended but it is one of the remedies that was once used, together with even more frightening methods, to 'bring back the hair'.

Another recipe for making the hair grow which is said to have been in use since the time of the Pharaohs in Egypt is to 'Seethe (boil) the leaves of the withy (willow) in oil and lay them where the hair is wanting'! Or, just to make you smile, for I am sure that no bald man would ever be vain or foolish enough to try it in these enlightened times, one old suggestion was to 'take cow-dung and the old soles of boots and burn them to powder in a new earthen pot fast stopped [tightly lidded] and then mingle the powder with raw honey to make an ointment thereof to anoynt thine head, covering it with a leather cap for nine days'.

Honey is often recommended for baldness, for external rather than the far less messy and probably far more efficacious internal use.

But neither a tendency towards early

baldness nor prematurely greying hair need detract from a healthy and attractive appearance. Some of the most tough and virile-looking men are bald, and indeed, as we all know, some young actors and film stars actually have their heads shaved thus to add to their beauty! Many young women, too, have their hair bleached and then tinted grey, so there is no longer any need to regard either of these problems as an ageing feature.

A really sad condition of baldness is when adolescents, usually for no obvious reason at all, suddenly start suffering from patchy hair-loss and baldness, or what is known as *Alopecia areata*, and suffer from unhappiness or acute self-consciousness because of it. They can be helped, as indeed anyone with hair-troubles can, by living on a high vitamin/fresh fruit/raw vegetable diet in which the carbohydrate intake is kept low, and by getting plenty of rest and freedom from stress. There are also external hair tonics to encourage the growth of new hair (see Therapeutic Index) and special shampoos made from Soap-bark Tree tincture instead of any other kind of soap.

The same treatment applies to those who suffer from dandruff or scurf, an abundance of which may easily be the forerunner of loss of hair. Do remember that both conditions are more easily coped with if the hair is kept short.

Greasy hair, from which so many people seem to suffer, will often benefit from a change to a better diet, especially one free from animal fats but also including plenty of fresh fruit and salad plants. Greasy hair needs more shampooing with herbal hair preparations than hair which is dry and brittle – a condition which seems to arise more and more as hair colour fades, or in menopausal or post-menopausal times.

To those of us who suffer from it, the latter state is often more difficult to cure than the former, but the external use of light plant oils and the inclusion of such commodities as Sunflower, Almond or Sesame oils as a dietary addition, as well as non-oily herbs like Parsley, Marigold, Nettles and Comfrey whenever there is an opportunity to use them raw, can help greatly. All these herbs are what I call 'inside and outside' remedies – useful both internally and externally!

The careful application of many different plant oils – according to the state of your purse, for many have to be imported and are now very expensive – can help dry hair very much. They range from Castor oil which is the heaviest, through Olive oil to the solid-when-cold Coconut oil or even Eucalyptus, which is a beneficial hair oil for those who do not mind its strong smell.

There is also Lavender oil which is delicious but very costly, as is the light Almond oil or even the cheaper Flax or Linseed oil (by which the old horsemen set such store for their fine animals' coats), or Green (elder) oil which can be very difficult to buy (but see page 27 for instructions for making). The choice is yours, but go lightly with whichever oil you decide upon or you will have to resort to the Victorian antimacassars again. Remember that a little oil, properly brushed or massaged into the head and scalp, goes a long way.

Cosmetic history and herbals through the ages show that women, and even men during some periods of history, have never been satisfied with the colour of their own hair, so that vegetable dyes, tints, rinses and powders have been used.

Henna, the hair dye of the Arabs even in biblical days (translated into the Hebrew 'Kopher' or 'Copher' and into 'Camphire' in the Song of Solomon), has always, it seems been first favourite, but unless it is used very carefully, it does give the hair an unnaturally strong reddish colour.

As this book shows, there are other milder, cheaper, easily obtainable herbs which can be used if you are not satisfied with the colour of your hair, but be wary of putting any dark solutions you may make, even from ordinary Tea or Walnut husks, or Sage, straight on to freshly washed and very absorbent hairs. Remember that any startling colours can take a long time to grow out!

Brightening rinses can be made from Chamomile for 'those who have fair hair that they would like to be fairer' by brewing a 'tea' with two teaspoonsful of the herb to a pint of boiling water. After cooling, experiment carefully with the solution on a strand of hidden hair before toppling the jugful over your head, as this could be too strong for some people. Chamomile tea, made with one teaspoonful of herb to a pint of boiling water and then carefully cooled, makes a safe rinse for children's hair, or even a shampoo if enough shredded Castile soap is added to make the liquid gently frothy.

Fortunately, we no longer need the

enormous number of herbal hair lotions, potions, powders, pommades and ointments with which our ancestors used to disguise their long unwashed locks. Then antiseptic herbs had to play a very real part in helping to keep their matted hair 'free of vermin', as well, no doubt, as from 'smelling sour'. But I hope you will see from this book that the basic use of herbs for helping hair to be at its best, or to regain health, still remains, even though hair care in general is now much simpler.

ALMOND
(Prunus dulcis)

Almond trees are best known in Northern European gardens because of their delightful, early pale pink blossom which appears before the leaves, sometimes as early as February. Their fruit-setting is only sporadic in cooler countries and edible oil-producing Almonds have to be imported.

Basically, there appear to be two commercially-grown varieties, the Sweet Almond and the Bitter Almond and for internal, and indeed external purposes the oil from the former is preferable. Strangely enough, although products from Bitter Almonds are now excluded from all medicinal use in this country because of their poisonous properties, they are still, as far as I know, allowed to be used by confectioners. They and Peach-nut kernels both contain a glucoside, Amygdalin, which is certainly harmful internally and does not exist at all in Sweet Almond.

The Almond provides a light lubricating oil which is preferable to the heavier Olive oil and is very useful for nourishing the scalp. A thorough massage 'right down to the roots of the hair' the night before a shampoo will do much to improve lifeless, dull, dry, scurfy (and what is dandruff but scurf?) hair.

After this massage the head should be wrapped in a warmed towel so that the oil can soak well in and if possible (and

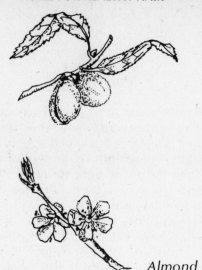

Almond

especially before a perm) kept wrapped up all night.

It is rather amusing to note that Macassar oil of which the Victorians were so fond (and I had never realized that the now despised chairback coverings known as 'antimacassars' were used to stop greasy heads from parting with their oil directly on to the upholstery) was made from Almond oil which was frequently scented with Cassia oil and coloured with the red dye from the Alkanet root.

Almond oil, according to old herbal literature, was often 'adulterated' by the addition of Teel, or Gingalee, oil, known to us as Sesame oil (see page 45), which our ancestors found fault with, but which we, realizing Sesame's virtues, should not worry about nowadays.

ARNICA
(Arnica montana)

Arnica is included in some herbal shampoos and has the reputation of being excellent for promoting hair growth. To me, this mountain 'Accident Plant' is a magic herb, providing a wonderful remedy for bruises, sprains and other muscular troubles when used externally, in diluted tincture form. Incidentally, it should never be applied when the skin is broken, and should always be used cold.

As hair can be called part of the skin – or perhaps it might be said to be an outgrowth

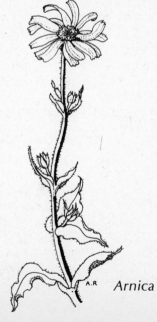

Arnica

of the skin, like the nails – it is not surprising that Arnica, which is such a vital and stimulating herb, is so helpful to healthy hair growth.

I have known cases when the hair has been in a poor state after severe illness, great anxiety or nervous shock – as well as after long courses of antibiotics have been prescribed – when hair tonic with Arnica in it has been of much value.

Now that the Trade Descriptions Act is well in force in Britain, of course, the herbal contents displayed, or even portrayed, on shampoo or hair-tonic packets (provided they are not pictures of purely imaginary plants), have to be included in their contents. So if your hair needs 'conditioning' look out for the name 'Arnica' or a picture of the handsome, yellow, daisy-shaped flower (which seems to be very difficult to grow) next time you buy a preparation for the care of your hair.

BAYBERRY or BAY-RUM TREE
(Pimenta acris)

There seems to have been some confusion among older herbalists as to the source of Bay-rum as there is another Bayberry tree *(Myrica cerifera)* as well, of course, as the Bay-laurel tree. The last, to add to the difficulty in sorting out these plants, provides 'Oil of Bays' which was used, and possibly still is, to alleviate the pain from bad bruises and sprains.

However, to the best of my knowledge, it is the West Indian Bayberry, also known as 'Wild Cinnamon', Jamaica Pepper-tree or *Pimenta acris*, from which the basic ingredient of the famous old hair tonic has always been obtained.

The Bay-rum tree used to be known as *Eugenia pimento*, thus showing its relationship to the Clove *(Eugenia aromatica)*. *Pimenta acris* are grown in groves, with the Allspice-bush *(Pimenta officinalis)* and the fruits of both are dried and then powdered down for the composite clove/nutmeg/cinnamon-flavoured spice known as Allspice.

But Bay-rum is made by the leaves from *Pimenta acris* tree being distilled in rum to produce a hair application with both fragrant and tonic virtues.

It will be useful for those who suffer from greasy hair and need a spirit-based, scalp-stimulating lotion to help them to control their locks!

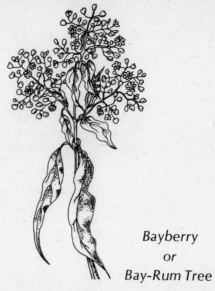

Bayberry

or

Bay-Rum Tree

I should guess that it was even more popular as a hair-cleanser in the days before showers and sprays were so frequently installed in bathrooms, when hair-washing was not as simple an operation as it is now. But Bay-rum hair lotions are still in great demand and still make useful and harmless applications which are said to help those with dandruff.

BIRCH
(Betula pendula)

Young Birch leaves and green twig-shoots contain a high percentage of vitamin C, an element which is essential to our diets and health, and encourages the strong and renewed growth of the hair.

Rudolf Steiner, described variously as a religious nature philosopher, mystic and seer, left indications when he died earlier this century about many valuable plants as sources of vital importance to increased 'oneness', and therefore well-being, with the natural world. Birch was one of them, and the

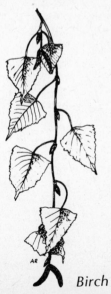

Birch

Swiss pharmacists who carry on his medicinally therapeutic work in their pure and delightful herbal preparations make much use of this plant.

Modern herbalists are also indebted to the Red Indians for handing on their knowledge about the attributes of Birch which has been traditionally used in spring tonics as well as for making a herbal tea to help rheumaticky or arthritic sufferers for generations. It was the Red Indians who extolled its virtues when an infusion of leaves was prepared to use as a scalp cleanser and stimulator of hair-growth.

This is the first of what I call 'inside and out' herbs to be mentioned in this book. Try a drink of Birch-leaf tea, sweetened with honey if you prefer it, and also use it, without the sweetening, to comb and brush through your hair as an invigorating, astringent and cleansing lotion.

BURDOCK
(Arctium lappa)

It may be surprising to find such a common wayside plant included in herbs 'recommended for healthy hair', but this strong plant, already useful in diet and as a herbal preparation in a variety of ways, supplies seeds from which a fluid extract is prepared, and this is invaluable for the skin, including the scalp.

The seeds are oily and most helpful to the glands of the hair, which are of two kinds, those that produce natural oil (the sebaceous glands) to keep the hair pliable and glossy, and the sometimes overfunctioning sweat-glands on the head.

Look out for pictures of the Burdock among the herbs used in shampoos, or the name Burdock in the list of ingredients, for this plant ought to be included in any that are offered specifically for dry hair. More people seem to suffer from this than any other hair disorder, especially as they get older and their hair starts losing its colour.

There are, of course, plenty of other plant oils available (see Almond, Lavender, Rosemary, Sesame, and Sunflower in this book) but Burdock seeds provide one that is very easily assimilated by the skin and can be taken internally too, if you care to collect the seed to grow on as winter 'sprouters' and then eat the baby plants as sandwich-fillers or in salads. The heads of hooked seeds can be

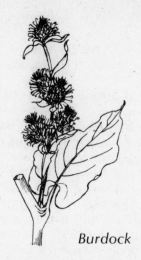

Burdock

gathered from hedgerows and roadsides in
the autumn, when indeed they often stick to
walkers' clothing and dog's coats as they
brush past them.

'Sprouting' seeds of different kinds (see
also Alfalfa, in *Herbs and Fruit for Vitamins*, in
this series) is easy, but it is as well to keep the
different species separate as their
germination rates vary. Any useful seeds can
be grown – after careful washing to remove
dirt and in some cases their outer skins – in
jars covered with muslin lids. The jars only
need rinsing out with clean water twice a day,
when the water should be strained off
through the muslin lid. If they are kept in a
warm room they germinate quickly and
provide vitamin-filled and mineral-rich salad
in the winter when other growing plant food
is scarce.

COMFREY
(Symphytum officinale)

Comfrey is one of our most healing and useful medicinal herbs. It contains – mainly in its roots – the crystalline substance *allantoin* which is used to promote the growth of fresh tissue in both internal and external ulceration. This was not really recognized until this century although older, non-analytical herbalists had always extolled the use of the plant for making 'plasters' from its mucilaginous leaves to apply to wounds, burns and even broken bones.

Culpeper realized its virtues, saying: 'A syrup made thereof is very effectual in inward hurts, and the distilled water for the same purpose also, and for outward wounds or sores in the fleshy or sinewy parts of the body ...'

Young Comfrey leaves, hairy as they may seem, can be eaten in salads, or cooked, very lightly, to make a palatable green vegetable which is thought not only to act as a tonic, but also to help those with poor circulation and 'poverty of blood'.

Country people often used to 'force' the shoots of Comfrey, and this is still done with Sea Kale and Chicory to provide tasty, tender and blanched vegetables. I found a plant early last Spring which had had a light pile of damp hay over it during the winter. It was very blanched and I took some etiolated shoots home and cooked them. I found them

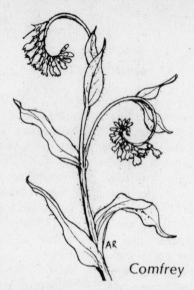

Comfrey

pleasant as soon as I had got used to their somewhat unusual taste.

Comfrey, as can be imagined from its high mucilaginous content, is one of the demulcent, or soothing, herbs and this is partly why those with coarse, dry hair often find that there is an improvement after they have added this herb to their diets. It seems to help them faster if they eat it raw, chopped in salads. There is often a marked improvement in the condition of the skin, too, and 'those with the acne', as a nineteenth-century herbalist wrote, 'especially if there are clusters of little pustules at the top of the forehead, or behind the ears, growing into where the roots of the hair begin, or again in eyebrows or the mustache, seem to benefit greatly.'

ELDER
(Sambucus nigra)

Elder has always been so generally useful to man since he discovered the virtues of its leaves, flowers, young shoots, pith, berries and even bark that it frequently takes up several pages of a big herbal!

Be that as it may. Here I shall simply mention that a herbal dye for fading hair can be made from the berries. This needs extremely careful application or you will find yourself with dark purple tresses, so dilute any berry-juice if you try it, to see how it 'takes' on your hair, and select a hidden strand to test it for the first time.

The famous Green Oil (also known as 'Oil of Swallows', and I have no indication whatsoever why it got this name) was made from Elder leaves and has been used, sometimes scented with more fragrant herbs, through the ages. It can be made at home by boiling one part of crushed Elder leaves with three parts of Linseed or Flax oil. The strained product makes a safe preparation to apply, with discretion, to the hair. When it is made commercially, dye is added to make it greener, but there is no need to colour it artificially for home use.

The old horsemen, full of superstitions as well as of practical knowledge, set much store on this 'Oil of Swallows' for keeping their animals' coats in perfect condition. They, of course, gave it internally (in bran mashes) in

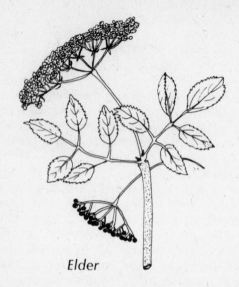

Elder

their various and often rather drastic medicines, but one I knew as an extremely old man still kept a dusty bottleful on his kitchen mantelpiece, with which he would often smear his bushy eyebrows and then, rubbing a few drops between his hands, would rub them lightly over his still thick hair. 'We used to polish their coats up a bit,' he told me, 'with this green Elder oil, before we put them into shows. Had to do it carefully, mind you, only a little like, or it might have come off on the judges' hands.'

Elder, incidentally, has a pleasing old reputation as 'the medicine chest of country people'. Evelyn dubbed it 'a catholicon against all infirmities whatever'.

When the plant is in flower the flat heads of the hay-scented creamy blooms can be used to make a delicious hair rinse. A most refreshing and scalp-invigorating final rinse can be made by putting two or three blooms in a big jug and then half filling it with boiling water. This can be topped up with cold water after they have seethed for a few minutes. The flowers are then strained off.

KELP
(Various seaweeds, including *Fucus* spp. &
Laminaria spp. in Europe and others from
other parts of the world.)

At times during our lives, especially after
periods of extra tension, or long illnesses and
weakness, our bodies often seem to be crying
out for something in the way of nutriment
that we are not taking in in our ordinary day-
by-day diet. These deficiencies often show up
in the state of our hair. Dry, brittle, rapidly
fading or, worst of all, falling hair is
frequently the external 'barometer' of our
condition.

The old horsemen always knew when their
horses were out of condition by the feel and
appearance of their coats. And we, whether
you like it or not, would do well to realize
that our hair too often reflects our physical
and mental state.

Vitamins, now that we know more about
their actions, are becoming easier to replace
naturally, but there are other essential diet
commodities that are not so well known yet,
although they may be offered in synthetized
forms by some medical practitioners. Many of
these mineral elements are easily obtained,
naturally, from Kelp.

Kelp is made from brown seaweeds which
were the first recognized source of iodine
and other important trace elements. It will
frequently provide 'the final link in the
balanced diet' because 'sea plants grow in a

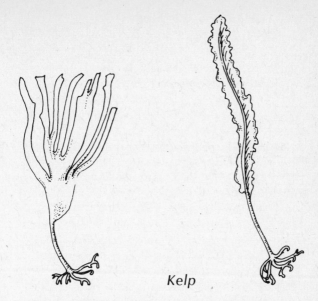

Kelp

mineral-rich medium', as Dr Jarvis said.

Kelp tablets are easy to take and a little careful experimentation will soon show you how few will 'do the trick'.

Some enthusiasts make their own Kelp-added salt by milling fresh 'greens' which include Nettle leaves, Shepherd's Purse leaves and young fruits (which are peppery rather than salty), and a Tansy leaf (which is bitter), together with other herbs, then adding the result to an equal amount of Kelp powder to use as a regular table condiment.

LAVENDER
(*Lavendula vera* and *Lavendula spica*)

Oil of Lavender is obtained only from the flowers and their spike-stalks and is expensive to buy. It is worth indulging occasionally in a small bottle of it from a reputable herbalist, for it goes a very long way when used carefully. But it is perfectly possible, if you are lucky enough to grow your own, to make the dried flowers into lavender 'bags', even adding the young leaf tips once they have been shredded, to use in hair-rinsing water.

A friend of mine runs up strips of 2-inch (5-cm), three-sided muslin square bags, side by side, like a long row of large tea-bags, on her sewing machine. She fills each while they are still in the piece, with a heaped teaspoonful or so of the flowers, shakes them well down and then machines along the top. Then the little bags are cut up, stored in a dry place until needed and infused, in the usual way, for hair-rinsing waters. (This method, of course, can be used for making herbal tisanes-sachets of many kinds).

The oil itself need only be applied to freshly washed hair before it is brushed. It has the reputation of 'sorting knots and tangles' and when rubbed with the finger-tips into the scalp acts as a stimulating and antiseptic lubricant. Its fragrance always seems to excite more comment than any other for everyone recognizes Lavender with its delicious summer scent.

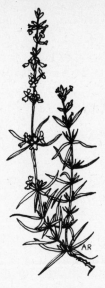

Lavender

English Lavender is still supposed to have the finest fragrance of all, although much of the commercially-prepared oil comes from the European Spiked Lavender *(L.spica)*, a coarser plant providing more oil quantatively speaking, but, so connoisseurs say, of lesser quality. However, curiously enough, it is this oil which is particularly good 'for promoting the growth of weakly, or falling hair'.

LEMON
(Citrus linonum)

It would be unthinkable to write a book about Herbs for Healthy Hair without mentioning Lemons. Not only do people with the most beautiful hair frequently acknowledge that they add a few drops of fresh lemon-juice to their first and last drinks of water every morning and evening, but they also, I have discovered, save their lemon rinds to add to their final hair rinses, as well as to the water in which they wash their brushes and combs.

When I was a child, my mother used to tell me to shut my eyes while she poured the last rinse containing lemon juice and the boiled rinds over my head. Then she would feel my hair and say : 'Nothing gets it more completely free from soap. Listen!' and she would rub a few hairs between her fingers, 'You can hear it squeak!'

I see now that one shampoo manufacturer who has put a lemon-scented product on the market advertises it as getting your hair 'Squeak-clean'.

I came across a recipe in a French chemist's Victorian repertory for *'Pomade contre L'Alopecie'*. It contained a dram of fresh lemon juice, and of course the fruit is frequently recommended for baldness or Alopecia. It looks as if there may be a connection between a vitamin-lack and this distressing symptom for which more and

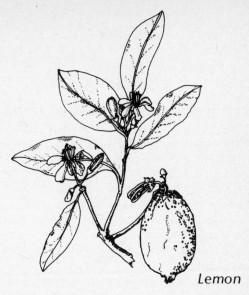

Lemon

more causes are being suggested. Alopecia,
by the way, is only another word for
'baldness' which may mean that the hair is
falling out in patches, a state which
sometimes, as I have mentioned, occurs in
adolescence as well as in later life, at times of
poor health, or of great anxiety or
unhappiness.

MARIGOLDS
(Calendula officinalis)

Many old herbals give lists of plants that were used through the ages for the skin and the hair, and Marigolds, with their 'pleasant bright and shining yellow flowers, the which do close at the setting downe of the sunne, and do spread and open againe at the sunne rising', frequently top these lists.

They were also used for ointments, plasters, lotions, potions (even love-potions), pommades, pomatums, and hair-fixers too, both for men and for women, but especially the latter perhaps, for: 'Of marygold we learn that Sunne use to make theyr heyr yellow with the floure of this herbe, not beying content with the naturall coloure which God hath given to them.'

Other herbalists have recommended the plants' leaves as cures for 'boyles and other suppurations on the head' or to 'heal cuts and wounds met with by falling head first from the horse'!

Marigold petals were not the only yellow ones used as a dye–those from the tall Mullein plant, and sometimes yellow Corn Marigolds or even the now rare Yellow Anthemis were frequently employed by those who wanted to be blonder than they were.

Modern herbalists still used Marigolds as wound healers, whether for the head or any other part of the body. Half a teaspoonful of Marigold tincture to a cup of cold water

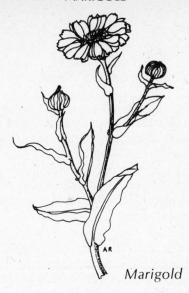

Marigold

makes a splendidly refreshing and antiseptic application which promotes the growth of healthy hair if used regularly for scalp massage. If you infuse a small handful of young leaves, buds and stems as well as a few flowers in a jugful of boiling water and leave this to cool down before using it as a rinse, it also acts as a slight setting-lotion.

Apart from massaging various oils *gently* into the head, I would suggest that Marigold, of all the hair herbs, is the most likely one to keep thinning hair from getting any thinner and even to help new hair grow to thicken the impoverished crop already there.

NETTLES
(Urtica dioica and *Urtica urens)*

During the past twenty years or so there has been a great deal of newly awakened interest in the medical and cosmetic use of herbs, as well as in more natural living. This, of course, has stemmed from more individuals finding out for themselves the various ways of using common herbs, almost up to commercial-level exploitation of them, and many shampoos that have been concocted under herbal guise are still based on detergent and extremely harsh cleansing agents.

Some, as I have said before, have delightful herb and flower labels to advertise them. Most of them produce green mixtures which smell of strong herbal tinctures, but it is wise to read their precise formulae before believing that you have bought yourself a beneficial hair-wash.

There are, however, several good British and European herbal cosmetic producers who offer beneficial and safe shampoos based on the mildest, purest soaps and including herbal extracts of such plants as Nettles.

Nettles have always been thought to be strengthening and stimulating to hair growth, but it is not essential to buy shampoos including this plant because Nettle 'tea', or a solution made by infusing a gloved handful of Nettles to a jugful of boiling water, can be used as a rinse. It will be noticed that the

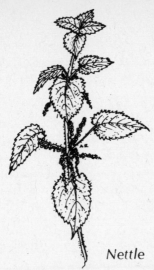

Nettle

Nettles colour the water as they 'brew', and people who are beginning to go grey claim that Nettle rinses keep their hair a good colour as well as leaving it 'lustrous and pliable'. Others say that Nettle rinses give lifeless, sun- or sea-bleached hair, or hair that is 'tired' after long illness, a real boost, and the herb comes very near the top of the list for those who suffer from dandruff.

If the smell of Nettles is still over-powering while your rinse is cooling add a few drops of oil of Lavender or even some Lemon or Orange peel. Personally, I find the 'green' smell of infused Nettles reminiscent of warm summer days when coloured butterflies flew round and over the stinging leaves looking for somewhere sheltered to deposit their eggs. The stinging-glands on Nettle leaves, by the way, are broken down directly the leaves are softened by boiling water.

ROSEMARY
(Rosmarinus officinalis)

Of all the many traditions associated with this aromatic and beautiful shrub, the best-known is possibly 'that it flourisheth best where the women ruleth the house!', followed by the saying that Rosemary never grows taller than the height of Christ. You will have to judge for yourselves whether either of these is strictly true or not, but remember, concerning the latter 'tall tale', that Rosemary is native to Mediterranean countries where it appears to sprawl and grow into a thicker, lower shrub in the hot sun than it does in northern areas.

Rosemary will, however, do well in many English gardens so long as it has the shelter of walls to keep off the worst of the northerly winds. It is reasonably tolerant to frost but falls of winter snow tend to break the brittle branches, and in long, cold winters, even in the southern counties, it also tends to lose its otherwise evergreen leaves. The saying has it that cuttings taken and planted on Good Friday, take readily, although I find that other days are also possible. I like to think that some of the Pilgrim fathers and mothers took Rosemary with them when they sailed over wide seas to fresh and hard lives in the New World.

Through the ages Rosemary has been the emblem of evergreen memories as well as appearing in garlands and bouquets on all

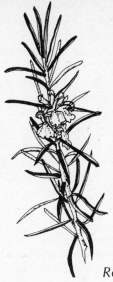

Rosemary

occasions. As Sir Thomas More said: 'It is the herb sacred to remembrance, and, thus to friendship', and it also, to go back to practicalities, has had a long association as a cleansing, fragrance-giving hair herb that is very 'medicinal to the head'.

The Countess of Hainault, Queen Philippa's mother, is thought to have sent the first sprig to her daughter in England with the instructions to use it as a repellant to moths, as a washing-water 'fragrancer', a promoter of lost appetite, a cure of gout, 'the cough', and a tooth-saving powder, when 'the Timber thereof' is 'burnt to coales'. She obviously expected her daughter to grow the plant on to provide herself with a real panacea!

Nowadays, herbalists use Rosemary as a stomachic and nervine plant and externally as an ingredient of hair-promoting shampoos, oils and lotions, knowing full well its reputation of preventing premature baldness and being a stimulant for increased activity of the 'hair-bulbs'.

Fresh or dried leaves can also be infused and used as a rinse or, made a little stronger, as a lotion to rub into the scalp to help scurfiness and dandruff and to prevent 'freshly curled hair from springing straight again if you have to go out in damp weather'.

14

SAGE
(Salvia officinalis)

As a countrywoman I believe that every gardener ought to grow Sage, even if, in towns, this is only possible in a window-box or flower-pot! It is an invaluable plant and can be used for a wide variety of purposes, from making a herbal tea for gargling (the plant has natural antiseptic properties) or for indigestion, or 'phlegm on the chest', to the perhaps less vital function of a 'mild deodorant'. And this is to say nothing of its culinary virtues.

A reasonably strong concoction, made from the leaves of Red Sage particularly, has been used throughout the ages as a hair dye. I have heard it called 'the Henna of the West'. The strength of the solution obviously depends on the amount of colour you want to give the hair but as the plant seems to have no toxic content when used externally, this is a harmless method of darkening naturally dark hair that is fading. A Sage rinse is also said to give pleasing highlights to any brunette.

Gerard, the Elizabethan herbalist, said that 'Sage is singularly good to colour and darken the hair as well as for the head and brain, it quickeneth the senses and memory, strengtheneth the sinews, restoreth health to those that have the palsy, and taketh away shaky tremblings of the members'. What more could anyone want?

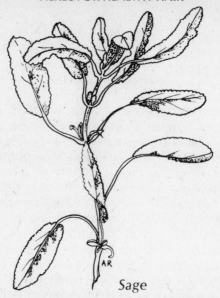

Sage

For a very dark Sage-tea rinse, it is possible to add 'powdered clove' and some people put a little borax into this solution. This is supposed to be excellent for staying falling hair, as well as promoting the growth of new hair.

It was another old herbalist who suggested that strong Sage tea 'takes away the smell of sour hair when brushed through carefully from root to tip every morning'. Sage is of course an astringent herb and would act as a scalp tonic for humans and a conditioner for animals' coats. I came across the following clue in a Victorian vetinary notebook: 'Always remember that sage chopped in a horse's feed gives him a better appetite while also improving the state of his coat be it staring, dull and lifeless'.

15

SESAME
(Sesamum indicum)

It is rather interesting to read in a Victorian botany book, that 'Many of the oriental nations look upon the Sesamum seeds as a hearty wholesome food, and express an oil from them not unlike, but inferior to, the oil of Almonds'.

How things change! Sesame oil is now regarded by natural food dietitians as vastly superior to that of many other plant oils as it contains lecithin which does not allow cholesterol to collect in the blood. It is also extremely pleasant to taste, as more and more people are finding out for themselves; its popularity is growing in the West and cakes and biscuits are now being made from whole Sesame seeds.

Sesame salt, or *gomasio* is popular too, especially by people interested in macrobiotic diets. It is made by roasting Sesame seeds with sea salt and then grinding them together. Once you have used *gomasio* and enjoyed its mild spiciness, you will not want to be without it. Sesame seeds are rich in vitamins and minerals, particularly iron, so that a creamy 'butter' or *tahini* made from them and obtainable in some health shops provides a valuable vegetable food as well.

Tahini is also used in that delicious though expensive 'sweet' *Halva* which is often on sale in health shops.

As Sesame seeds and the oil from them are

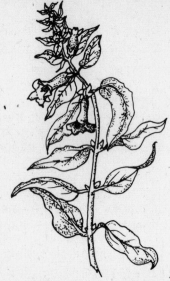

Sesame

so full of virtue for most people, including those who long to have glossy, healthy hair, they are a recommended addition to the diet. The seeds can be used in salads or as 'crispers' on top of bread or biscuits and cakes, and the expressed oil, of course, can be added to many 'raw food' meals.

It is also an excellent light hair oil and is used a great deal for this purpose in the East where it is scented with exotic flower perfumes. It seems particularly to suit those with coarse, dry, white hair, making it much more amenable to setting, or even taking a perm.

16

SOAP-BARK TREE
(Quillaja saponaria)

A tincture made from *Quillaja saponaria* is recommended in orthodox medical dictionaries as an ingredient in shampoos for those who are suffering from falling hair and incipient baldness.

The tree grows in South America, primarily in Chile, but other species of the same genus can be grown in areas where there are mild enough winters, even in this country. It has been suggested that the Soap-bark Tree is 'quite hardy enough to survive our winters and ripened cuttings will probably root if planted in the autumn'. As far as I know no one has had much success with it here or anywhere else in Northern Europe.

Quillaja saponaria was first brought to Britain as a botanical specimen in 1832 and it must have created a sensation when it was found how high the saponin content of its bark was. It is hardly surprising that the use of tincture made from this soapy bark is so frequently recommended in preference to the far harsher, often chemically or synthetically produced mixtures that are on sale in superficially attractive guise.

This tree is a member of the wing-seeded section of the Rose family and is an evergreen with toothed, oval, thick, leathery, shining-green leaves. It has white flowers that may grow singly at the tips of the branches or in clusters of three to five at a time. The Soap-

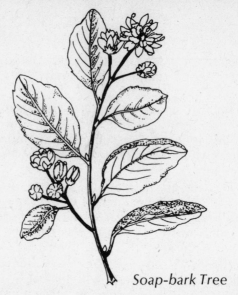

Soap-bark Tree

bark tree grows up to 50 or 60 feet (16-20 metres) high in its native country.

It is also known as the Panama Bark Tree, and Cullay, and the bark, which is very tough, dark and scentless is very astringent. As well as its soapy content it is full of scalp and hair-nourishing minerals, including calcium. Although it is now only used externally, for making shampoos for the hair and for cleaning materials, *Quillaja* was once used to make soft drinks foamy. The herb has been found to be harmful if taken internally, however, and this is now illegal. It has been, and probably still is, being used, in the correct dosage, by orthodox and homoeopathic medical practitioners. It should never be tried by amateurs.

The soap action of this tree bark is

comparable with that from our herbaceous Soapwort *(Saponaria officinalis)*. This makes a shampoo and cleaning agent for the most delicate of fabrics, a fact which was re-discovered earlier this century by Lady Meade-Fetherstonehaugh of Uppark, near Chichester in West Sussex. She found that a solution made from Soapwort could be used to clean ancient and valuable tapestries and hangings with far more safety than any other soap or cleaning preparation. It was even found to help these old fabrics to 'hold together' and it certainly brought out colours that appeared to have faded beyond all hope.

The Soap-bark tree in South America also provides cleaners with a safe solution for renovating the most fragile fabrics, so no wonder it is so good for the hair.

17

SOUTHERNWOOD
(Artemisia abrotanum)

This beautiful, green-grey fine-leaved aromatic herb has many popular names, the best-known among them probably being 'Old Man', or 'Garde Robe' or the delightful 'Appleringie' or 'Lad's Love'. The last points to one of the plant's oldest reputations which is that it encourages hair to grow on boys' beardless faces, when, or just as, in obvious fact, they are coming up to puberty.

It is likely that its quality, quoted in ancient times, of being able to 'draw forth splinters and thorns out of the flesh', as well as 'to burst all manner of pimples' was quickly transferred into helping the first reluctant and often acne-accompanied hairs through their young complexions.

But Culpeper says too that 'the ashes [of Southernwood] thereof, mingled with old sallet oyl, halps those what have their hair fallen and are bald causing the hair to grow again, either on the head or on the beard'.

My old country neighbour, who had a fine head of white hair, used to rub a leafy branch-tip of 'Old Man', which grew in his garden, between his fingers, after spitting on them, and rub it on to his eyebrows which were bushy and a pleasing dark grey. He maintained that the plant helped them to stay that way and an infusion made from this herb used as a final rinse certainly has the reputation of helping to give fresh life to greasy, dark, lank hair.

Southernwood, with other aromatic herbs, was one of the fragrant herbs in the various pomades, hair-powders and compounds used by our ancestors to embellish their locks. Frequent hair-washing must have been more difficult for them than it is for us, and it seems likely that many of the naturally antiseptic herbs that they used for their hair must have saved many of them from premature baldness as well as from having too many infestations of head parasites.

I pick and dry the leafy branch-tips of this herb in July or August when it is at its most fragrant, spreading them out on the sun-room floor on sheets of paper for a few days. When they are dry, I crumble them down to powder which I often mix in with my home-

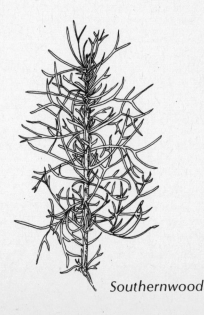

Southernwood

made shampoos (finely-shredded Castile soap, a few drops of oil of Lavender and usually any other aromatic or deliciously scented herbs, that I have ready) and add to rinsing-waters all through the winter. The physical effect, as well as the psychological uplift, is most refreshing, especially during the shortest and darkest days.

18

SUNFLOWER
(Helianthus annuus)

There are so many vegetable oils that, if carefully used, can help to keep the hair healthy – including Eucalyptus, Coconut (which is also very good for eyebrows and eye-lashes when applied with great care), Soya, (another 'inside and out' herb as Soya beans provide extremely nourishing protein-providing food) as well as the traditional Olive oil, and that of Lavender (see page 32), Sesame (see page 45), and Almond (see page 15) – that the numerous qualities of Sunflower oil can be forgotten.

But there are herb users who put Sunflower at the top of the hair-helping list, saying that eating the delicious seeds will improve the texture and the look of dry and lifeless hair. Indeed Ben Charles Harris, in his book *Eat the Weeds*, says that after eating a good handful every day he noticed that his hair became more oily, 'where before it had been dry and brittle'.

I would echo that sentiment and also the fact that he found that Sunflower seeds helped his eyesight very much too, for after eating his handful of them for only two weeks he became aware of a 'definite and most unbelievable change', as the strain and ache of his eyes almost disappeared.

Sunflower seeds are about 50 per cent oil, which is comparable to the amount in Olives. This is used in the manufacture of some

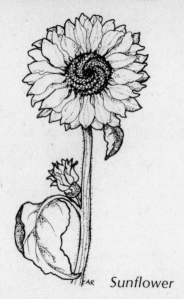

Sunflower

vegetable oil margarines (which are better for you than butter as they provide a source of unsaturated fatty acids). Sunflower oil is extremely rich in vitamin A and B and also helps to reduce, or certainly does not add to, the cholesterol level in the blood.

Many people use this oil for dressing salads and keep another small bottleful to apply to their hair, hoping perhaps to help themselves towards the 'glossy, dark locks of the American Indians' who are traditionally known to have used it lavishly.

The tall, handsome Sunflower, can grow, even in such variable climates as Britain and Northern Europe, up to 15 feet (5 metres) high during its summer life. As can be seen from its Latin name, it is only an annual, and has a stout stem and many leaves. The flowers, which are yellow, sun-like and about the size of soup plates, nod towards the earth a little but follow the sun from east to west during its daily journey, as if they are trying to get the maximum benefit from its rays. It is interesting that more and better quality seeds are produced by Sunflowers that grow in warm, sunnier seasons and climates.

19

WATERCRESS
(Nasturtium officinale)

Watercress is, of course, to be eaten, not to be used as an external application. As much fresh, raw salad food as possible should be included in the daily diet, and Watercress can be used in a variety of ways.

Now that it is grown in special, unpolluted shallow beds in so many parts of the country, it is usually easy to get hold of it daily. As a source of vitamins (A, B, C, and E) and such valuable substances as iron and other mineral trace elements, as well as plenty of beautiful green chlorophyll, it is a good means of taking these hair-tonic ingredients into the system.

Watercress sandwiches, Watercress as a garnish, Watercress in green salads – in fact any way that you can think of eating this herb raw – are all helpful. Even for people who cannot manage to eat much bulk in salads, Watercress provides a concentrated mass of highly useful health-giving assets in an easily assimilable form.

Don't cook it! I do know what a delicious soup it makes, but what a waste of vitamins. Heat destroys, or at least lessens, the vitamin-content of fresh foods and the B-complex vitamins and vitamin C are soluble in water as well. If you must cook it, at least use very little water and keep and use the liquid after cooking.

Watercress has long been renowned as a

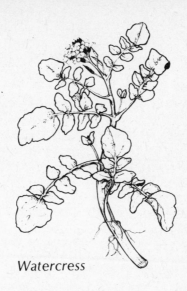

Watercress

skin herb, helping to 'clear the complexion' and keep it healthy in youth and old age. It is a most useful and good condition-maintaining herb for the elderly for whom the ancients suggested it as suitable for 'encouraging the wit and dispelling the lethargy'.

But do not forget, if Watercress is difficult to get in your district, that Landcress has many similar attributes and makes a tasty salad herb. This will grow, literally, on any patch of soil, or even in a window-box. The seed is obtainable from many seedsmen and after you have grown your first plant and let it mature, you need never be without it again as it scatters its seeds lavishly all around it.

20

YARROW
(Achillea millefolium)

Yarrow is a common wayside plant which grows in towns as well as in rural districts and has been popular through the ages, a fact which can be partly recognized from its long list of 'country names'. These include 'Soldiers', Woundwort', 'Carpenters' Weed', 'Staunchwort' (all of which denote its value as a vulnerary), but also perhaps its oldest, 'Baldwort'.

Yarrow 'stays the shedding of the hair, the head being bathed with the decoction of it' according to Culpeper, and to another herbalist it 'both beautifies and conditions the hair' if applied as a reasonably strong solution, together with the additon of an infusion of nettles (see page 38), which should then be brushed deeply through the hair for five minutes, 'every morning and night'.

Some care is necessary with these old suggestions as both Yarrow and Nettle are vital herbs and the solution should not be made too strong at first. An ounce (28g) of each herb to a pint (500ml) or even a pint and a half (750ml) of boiling water ought not to irritate the most sensitive scalp, but use your own commonsense and a good *bristle* brush – certainly not one with nylon or other manmade fibres in its make-up. The value of the stimulation from brushing the hair frequently comes under attack, and there are some

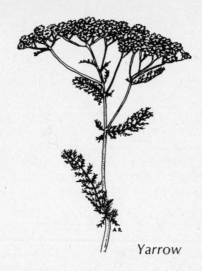

Yarrow

people with scant, thin hair who may find that they have to take it more easily.

Other herbs have been used to try to prevent falling hair, including Peach-leaves, Parsnip-root or seeds – $\frac{1}{4}$oz. (7g) to a cupful of vegetable oil, boiled together and strained when cool – and, for those suffering from dandruff, a 'strong tea made from the leaves and bark of the Willow tree'.

But, as I have tried to stress throughout this book, ninety-nine times out of a hundred the cause of falling hair (except in cases of hereditary baldness, severe illness, or some industrial' helmet, or hat-wearing cause) is governed to a great extent by its owner's general health and condition. Local measures can certainly be a help, but a healthy mind and body generally produces a healthy head of hair, so it is important to look to your diet, to take plenty of exercise *and* rest, and to do your best to rid yourself of unnecessary stress.

THERAPEUTIC INDEX

Acne, Comfrey, Marigold, Nettle (internally as a 'tea'), Southernwood, Watercress (internally).

Alopecia, see *Baldness*.

Antibiotics, see Arnica.

Antiseptic Plants, Arnica, Eucalyptus (see Introduction), Lavender, Lemon, Marigold, Rosemary, Sage, Southernwood.

Baldness, Kelp, Lemon, Marigold, Nettle, Parsnip and Peach-leaves (see Introduction), Rosemary, Sage, Soap-bark Tree, Southernwood, Willow (see Introduction and Yarrow), Yarrow.

Brushing lotions, Bay-rum, Birch, Burdock, Marigold, Nettle, Rosemary, Sage, Southernwood, Yarrow.

Curl-keeper, Rosemary.

Dandruff, see *Scurf*.

Dry Hair, Almond, Burdock, Kelp, Lavender, Rosemary, Sesame, Sunflower (and see *Hair oils*).

Greasy Hair, Bay-rum, Lemon, Southernwood (and see *Brushing lotions*).

Hair colourers, Chamomile (see Introduction), Elder, Marigold, Mullein (see Marigold), Nettle, Sage, Walnut (see Introduction).

Hair conditioners, Arnica, Birch, Elder, Kelp, Lavender, Lemon, Nettle, Rosemary, Sage, Southernwood, Watercress (internally).

Hair oils, Almond, Burdock, Elder, Eucalyptus (see Introduction), Lavender, Olive and

Linseed or Flax (see Introduction), Rosemary, Sesame, Sunflower.

Hair stimulants for growth, Arnica, Bay-rum, Birch, Lavender, Marigold, Nettle, Rosemary.

Hair tonics, Arnica, Bay-rum, Burdock, Elder, Kelp (internally), Lemon, Marigold, Nettle, Rosemary, Sage, Soap-bark tree, Southernwood, Sunflower seeds (internally), Watercress (internally).

Inside and Outside Herbs', Almond, Birch, Burdock, Comfrey, Elder, Lemon, Nettle, Sage, Sesame, Sunflower.

Rinses, (as 'teas'), Elder-flowers, Lavender, Lemon, Nettle, Marigold, Rosemary, Sage.

Scalp-massagers, see *Brushing lotions, Hair stimulants* and *Tonics.*

Scurf, Almond, Bay-rum, Lavender, Lemon, Nettle, Rosemary.

Setting lotion, Marigold (especially if buds are used).

Shampoos, Home-made Herbal Shampoo see Introduction, also Lemon, Marigold, Nettle, Rosemary, Sage, Soap-bark tree, Yarrow.

Untanglers of knots, Lavender and other 'light oils' e.g. Sesame.

Have you read these best selling ABOUT books?

ABOUT GINSENG

This book tells how ginseng has been used as a panacea for thousands of years in the East, describes its natural habitat and its cultivation throughout the world, and gives scientific evidence of its properties — especially its effect on the ageing process. The author reviews the different forms available and gives advice on how best to take it.

ABOUT VITAMINS

In this age of processed foods it is becoming increasingly more important to ensure that our diets provide us with an adequate supply of vitamins for the maintenance of good health. This book, an introduction to the subject of vitamins, clears away any misunderstandings that might exist, and tells the fascinating story of man's discovery of nature's keys to radiant health.

ABOUT RAW JUICES

The juices of fresh fruit and vegetables play a vital part in restoring and maintaining optimum health, and this book shows you how to select, prepare and use such life-giving and delicious drinks both for fortification against disease and for the specific treatment of certain ailments.

ABOUT GARLIC

Gives the historical background to this amazing herb, and shows how its miraculous healing powers can protect your health and assist the cure of many and varied complaints. The book also contains hints on the use of garlic in the kitchen, and recipes are included for garlic flavoured dishes.